FATTY LIVER AND CIRRHOSIS DIET COOKBOOK

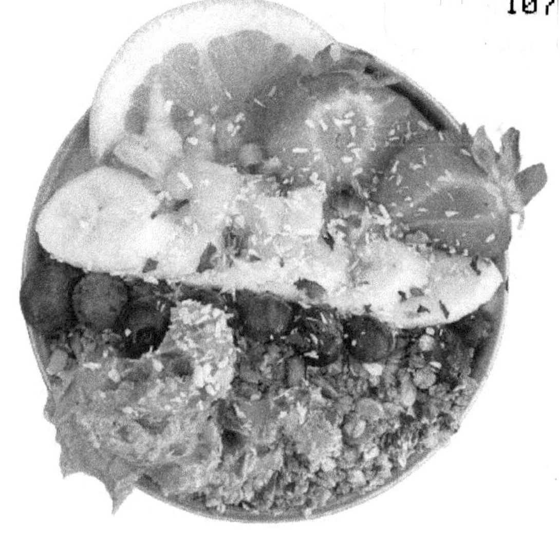

"Nutritious Recipes for a fatty liver and Cirrhosis Diet"

REGINA ANDERSON

Copyright © 2023 by Regina Anderson

DISCLAIMER

This cookbook is intended to provide general information and recipes.

The recipes provided in this cookbook are not intended to replace or be a substitute for medical advice from a physician.

The reader should consult a healthcare professional for any specific medical advice, diagnosis or treatment.

Any specific dietary advice provided in this cookbook is not intended to replace or be a substitute for medical advice from a physician.

The author is not responsible or liable for any adverse effects experienced by readers of this cookbook as a result of following the recipes or dietary advice provided.

The author makes no representations or warranties of any kind (express or implied) as to the accuracy, completeness, reliability or suitability of the recipes provided in this cookbook.

The author disclaims any and all liability for any damages arising out of the use or misuse of the recipes provided in this cookbook. The reader must also take care to ensure that the recipes provided in this cookbook are prepared and cooked safely.

The recipes provided in this cookbook are for informational purposes only and should not be used as a substitute for professional medical advice, diagnosis or treatment.

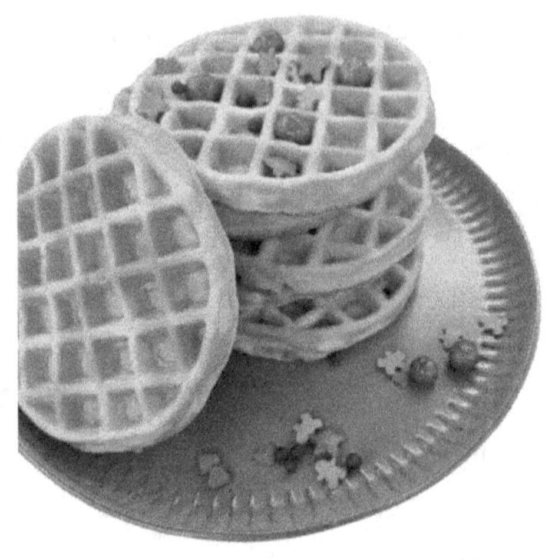

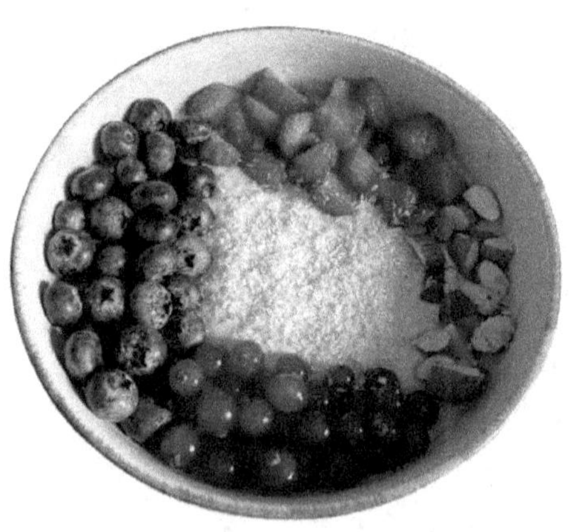

TABLE OF CONTENTS

INTRODUCTION

The liver is an important conductor in the complex symphony of body functions, coordinating activities that maintain life and energy.

But diseases like cirrhosis and fatty liver disease can interfere with this smooth operation, putting the liver under a lot of strain.

In response to these difficulties, following a unique diet turns into a calculated move that will both improve liver function and lessen the effects of these ailments.

A careful and encouraging meal plan is necessary for both cirrhosis, and fatty liver disease, which is characterized by the buildup of excess fat in liver cells.

A Fatty Liver and Cirrhosis Diet is more than just a recipe book, it's a map that points you in the direction of healthful decisions that may help with symptoms, improve liver function, and raise your quality of life.

The goal of this extensive dietary advice is to offer a clearer comprehension of the complex relationship between liver health and nutrition.

This book contains recipes that have been carefully chosen to meet the special dietary requirements of people with fatty liver disease and cirrhosis.

In addition to the tasty culinary creations, each meal features carefully chosen ingredients that assist liver regeneration, reduce inflammation, and help control weight.

Taking a holistic approach to starting this nutritional journey is necessary, understanding the relationship between nutrition, lifestyle, and general health.

Not only are you changing the way you eat, but you are also giving yourself the knowledge and resources you need to take an active role in your health journey when you follow the guidelines of the Fatty Liver and Cirrhosis Diet.

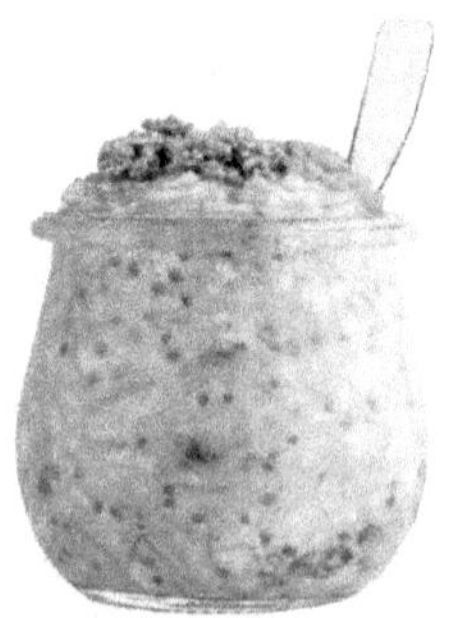

CHAPTER 1

9 BENEFITS OF EATING FATTY LIVER AND CIRRHOSIS DIET

1. **Decreased Liver Fat Accumulation:** One of the main concerns with fatty liver disease is the buildup of extra fat in the liver cells, which can be lessened with a diet that is properly chosen.

2. **Weight Control:** Adhering to a particular diet helps promote good weight control and lowers the chance of liver problems associated with obesity.

3. **Enhanced Insulin Sensitivity:** By improving insulin sensitivity, certain dietary options may help control blood sugar levels and maybe reduce the risk of type 2 diabetes.

4. **Reduction of Inflammation:** Anti-inflammatory foods are frequently the mainstay of a liver-friendly diet, which helps to reduce inflammation both in the liver and throughout the body.

5. **Support for Liver Regeneration:** Foods high in nutrients can supply the vital components needed for liver regeneration, accelerating the recovery process.

6. **Ideal Consumption of Nutrients:** The focus of a nutrient-dense diet for cirrhosis and fatty liver is to make sure the body gets the vitamins and minerals it needs for general health.

7. **Stabilized Blood Pressure:** Making certain dietary modifications, such cutting back on sodium, can help better control blood pressure and improve cardiovascular health in general.

8. **Promotes Detoxification:** Liver-friendly meals promote the liver's natural detoxification processes, which help the body rid itself of toxins. This results in enhanced detoxification.

9. **Better Digestive Health:** Eating foods high in fibre and easy to digest will help maintain gut health, which may help ease the discomfort that comes with liver disease-related digestive problems.

FOODS TO EAT AND AVOID ON A FATTY LIVER AND CIRRHOSIS DIET

13 FOODS TO EAT

1. **Fatty Fish:** Fatty fish, such as salmon, mackerel, and trout, are high in omega-3 fatty acids, which lower inflammation and promote liver health in general.

2. **Olive Oil:** Rich in beneficial monounsaturated fats, olive oil lowers cholesterol and has anti-inflammatory properties.

3. **Leafy Greens (Swiss Chard, Kale, Spinach):** Leafy greens, which are abundant in vitamins, minerals, and antioxidants, help to lessen oxidative stress and aid in liver detoxification.

4. **Avocado:** Packed with minerals and good fats, especially monounsaturated fats, it supports liver function.

5. **Walnuts:** Rich in antioxidants and omega-3 fatty acids, walnuts help keep the liver healthy and reduce inflammation.

6. **Berries (strawberries, blueberries):** Packed in antioxidants, these fruits protect the liver from oxidative damage and inflammation.

7. **Brussels sprouts and broccoli:** Brussels sprouts and broccoli are cruciferous vegetables that have nutrients that aid in the liver's detoxification activities.

8. **Turmeric:** Well-known for its anti-inflammatory qualities, turmeric can assist general liver function and lessen inflammation in the liver.

9. **Green Tea:** Rich in antioxidants, green tea has been linked to better liver function and a decrease in the formation of fat.

10. **Allicin:** Allicin, a substance found in garlic that has anti-inflammatory and antioxidant qualities, supports the health of the liver.

11. **Quinoa:** A complete grain that aids in weight management by encouraging fullness and offering fibre and protein.

12. **Sweet potatoes:** Rich in antioxidants, vitamins, and fibre, sweet potatoes are a part of a diet that is both liver-friendly and well-rounded.

13 FOODS TO AVOID

1. **Fried meals:** Fried meals include a lot of trans fats, which are bad for you and can cause inflammation and damage to your liver. Steer clear of deep-fried foods like fried chicken and French fries.

2. **Processed Meats:** Preservatives and additives are frequently found in processed meats. They also include a lot of saturated fats, which might aggravate liver inflammation. Lean, unprocessed meats are the better choice.

3. **Sugary Drinks:** Fruit juices and sodas are examples of sugary drinks that include a lot of added sugar. Limiting or avoiding these beverages is essential since fatty liver disease is associated with excessive sugar intake.

4. **Foods that have undergone extensive processing:** These foods frequently include unhealthy fats, preservatives, and additives. Eat whole, minimally processed foods to help maintain the health of your liver.

5. **White Bread and Pasta:** Refined carbs, such as those found in white bread and pasta, have the

potential to aggravate fatty liver disease by elevating blood sugar levels and causing weight gain.

6. **Over salted:** Consuming a lot of sodium can cause fluid retention and accelerate the development of cirrhosis. Reduce your salt intake by staying away from highly processed and salted foods.

7. **Alcohol:** One of the main causes of liver disease is alcohol. Alcohol should not be consumed by those with cirrhosis or fatty liver disease in order to protect their liver from additional damage.

8. **High-Fat Dairy:** Saturated fats are abundant in full-fat dairy products. To cut back on saturated fat consumption, go for low-fat or fat-free products.

9. **Red and Processed Meats:** Saturated fats included in red and processed meats can cause inflammation and damage to the liver. Choose lean protein sources such as fish, chicken, and plant-based substitutes.

10. **High-Fructose Corn Syrup:** Consuming foods and drinks high in fructose corn syrup can exacerbate fatty liver disease and insulin resistance. Examine product labels and select items that contain natural sweeteners sparingly.

CHAPTER 2

14-DAY MEAL PLAN

DAY 1

Breakfast: Smoothie with Low-sugar Yogurt, Fruits and Protein Powder

Lunch: Broiled Chicken with Roasted Potatoes

Dinner: Broccoli Quinoa Patties with Almond Butter

DAY 2

Breakfast: Wholewheat Waffle, Yogurt and Fresh Fruits

Lunch: Quinoa Salad with Edamame and Sweet Potatoes

Dinner: Roasted Vegetable Sandwich with Hummus

DAY 3

Breakfast: Overnight Steel-Cut Oat with Berries

Lunch: Veggie Toast with Hummus

Dinner: Curried Chickpea Wraps

DAY 4

Breakfast: Banana, Almond Chia Pudding

Lunch: Salmon with Roasted Vegetables

Dinner: Avocado Veggie Sandwich

DAY 5

Breakfast: Sprouted Grain Avocado Toast

Lunch: Grilled Turkey Sandwich with Cottage Cheese

Dinner: Grilled Fish Tacos with Avocados

DAY 6

Breakfast: Buckwheat Pancakes

Lunch: Baked Tilapia with Quinoa Pilaf

Dinner: Stir-Fried Shrimp and Vegetables

DAY 7

Breakfast: Tofu Scramble with Veggies

Lunch: Cauliflower Rice Bowl with Chickpeas and Spinach

Dinner: Quinoa and Roasted Vegetables

DAY 8

Breakfast: Beetroot and Nut Butter Smoothie Bowl

Lunch: Carrot and Couscous Soup

Dinner: Brown Rice Pilaf

DAY 9

Breakfast: Spicy Lentil Patties with Veggies

Lunch: Zucchini Noodles with Kale and Tomato Sauce

Dinner: Lentil Soup

DAY 10

Breakfast: Quinoa Porridge with Berries

Lunch: Lentil Tacos with Avocado

Dinner: Egg White Omelet

DAY 11

Breakfast: Smoothie with Low-sugar Yogurt, Fruits and Protein Powder

Lunch: Broiled Chicken with Roasted Potatoes

Dinner: Broccoli Quinoa Patties with Almond Butter

DAY 12

Breakfast: Wholewheat Waffle, Yogurt and Fresh Fruits

Lunch: Quinoa Salad with Edamame and Sweet Potatoes

Dinner: Roasted Vegetable Sandwich with Hummus

DAY 13

Breakfast: Overnight Steel-Cut Oat with Berries

Lunch: Veggie Toast with Hummus

Dinner: Curried Chickpea Wraps

DAY 14

Breakfast: Banana, Almond Chia Pudding

Lunch: Salmon with Roasted Vegetables

Dinner: Avocado Veggie Sandwich

CHAPTER 3

NUTRITIOUS RECIPES FOR A FATTY LIVER AND CIRRHOSIS DIET

BREAKFAST

Smoothie with Low-sugar Yogurt, Fruits, and Protein Powder

Preparation Time: 5 minutes

Serves: 1

Calories: 250 **Sugar:** 12g **Sodium:** 120mg

Ingredients:

1 cup low-sugar yogurt

1/2 cup mixed berries (blueberries, strawberries, raspberries)

1 scoop protein powder (low sugar)

1/2 banana

1/2 cup almond milk

Ice cubes (optional)

Method of Preparation:

1. Blend together almond milk, banana, protein powder, mixed berries, low-sugar yoghurt, and banana in a blender.
2. Mix until homogeneous.
3. If desired, add ice cubes and mix one more.
4. After pouring into a glass, savor!

Wholewheat Waffle, Yogurt, and Fresh Fruits

Preparation Time: 10 minutes

Serves: 1

Calories: 300 **Sugar:** 15g **Sodium:** 180mg

Ingredients:

1 wholewheat waffle)

1/2 cup low-fat yogurt

Mixed fresh fruits (e.g., berries, sliced kiwi, banana)

1 tablespoon honey (optional)

Method of Preparation:

1. Toast the wholewheat waffle per the directions on the package or to your own taste.
2. Cover the waffle with a layer of low-fat yoghurt.
3. Sprinkle some fresh fruit on top.
4. If desired, drizzle with honey.

Overnight Steel-Cut Oat with Berries

Preparation Time: 5 minutes (plus overnight soaking)

Serves: 1

Calories: 280 **Sugar:** 8g **Sodium:** 80mg

Ingredients:

1/2 cup steel-cut oats

1/2 cup mixed berries (strawberries, blueberries)

1 tablespoon chia seeds

1/2 cup low-fat milk or plant-based milk

1/2 teaspoon vanilla extract

1 teaspoon honey (optional)

Method of Preparation:

1. Steel-cut oats, mixed berries, chia seeds, milk, and vanilla essence should all be combined in a container or bowl.
2. Give it a good stir, making sure the oats are well covered by the liquid.
3. Refrigerate overnight with a cover on.
4. Stir well in the morning, then garnish with honey, if you wish.

Banana, Almond Chia Pudding

Preparation Time: 10 minutes + chilling time

Serves: 2

Calories: 250 **Sugar:** 15g **Sodium:** 80mg

Ingredients:

2 ripe bananas

1/4 cup chia seeds

1 cup almond milk

1/4 cup sliced almonds

Method of Preparation:

1. Blend almond milk and ripe bananas in a blender until smooth.
2. Transfer the mixture of bananas into a bowl and mix in the chia seeds.
3. After putting the mixture in the fridge for two hours or overnight, the chia seeds will absorb the liquid and thicken into a pudding-like consistency.
4. Serve with sliced almonds on top.

Sprouted Grain Avocado Toast

Preparation Time: 10 minutes

Serves: 2

Calories: 200 **Sugar:** 1g **Sodium:** 150mg

Ingredients:

2 slices sprouted grain bread

1 ripe avocado

Salt and pepper to taste

Optional toppings: cherry tomatoes, radish slices, or microgreens

Method of Preparation:

1. Toast the slices of sprouted grain bread according to your preference.
2. Mash the ripe avocado and season with salt and pepper while the bread is browning.
3. Over the toasty bread slices, equally distribute the mashed avocado.
4. Add your preferred optional toppings on top.

Buckwheat Pancakes

Preparation Time: 20 minutes

Serves: 4

Calories: 220 **Sugar:** 4 **Sodium:** 200

Ingredients:

1 cup buckwheat flour

1 tablespoon coconut sugar

1 teaspoon baking powder

1/4 teaspoon salt

1 cup almond milk

1 large egg

1 tablespoon coconut oil, melted

Fresh berries for topping (optional)

Method of Preparation:

1. Buckwheat flour, coconut sugar, baking powder, and salt should all be combined in a big bowl.
2. Melted coconut oil, egg, and almond milk should all be combined in a different bowl.
3. Mixing until just mixed, pour the wet components into the dry ingredients.
4. Over medium heat, preheat a nonstick skillet or griddle. For each pancake, transfer 1/4 cup of batter onto the griddle.
5. Cook until surface bubbles appear, then turn and continue cooking until golden brown on the other side.
6. If preferred, top with fresh berries and serve.

Tofu Scramble with Veggies

Preparation Time: 20 minutes

Serves: 2

Calories: 250 **Sugar:** 2g **Sodium:** 300mg

Ingredients:

Firm tofu

Bell peppers

Spinach

Cherry tomatoes

Olive oil

Turmeric

Salt and pepper to taste

Method of Preparation:

1. Crumble the tofu after pressing it to get rid of extra water.

2. After softening the bell peppers, add the tomatoes and spinach.

3. Stir in the turmeric, salt, pepper, and crumbled tofu. Cook until well heated.

Beetroot and Nut Butter Smoothie Bowl

Preparation Time: 10 minutes

Serves: 1

Calories: 300 **Sugar:** 15g **Sodium:** 150mg

Ingredients:

Cooked beets

Banana

Almond butter

Greek yogurt

Chia seeds

Almond milk

Method of Preparation:

1. Smoothly blend cooked beets, banana, Greek yoghurt, almond milk, and almond butter.

2. Pour into a bowl and garnish with banana slices and chia seeds.

Spicy Lentil Patties with Veggies

Preparation Time: 30 minutes

Serves: 4 **Calories:** 180 **Sugar:** 4g **Sodium:** 200mg

Ingredients:

Cooked lentils

Carrots

Onions

Garlic

Cumin and coriander

Whole wheat breadcrumbs

Egg (or flaxseed egg for a vegan option)

Method of Preparation:

1. Garlic, onions, and carrots should be sautéed until soft. Add to blended lentils.

2. Stir in the egg, breadcrumbs, coriander, and cumin. Shape into patties, then cook.

Quinoa Porridge with Berries

Preparation Time: 25 minutes

Serves: 3

Calories: 220 **Sugar:** 8g **Sodium:** 100mg

Ingredients:

Quinoa

Almond milk

Mixed berries

Honey or maple syrup

Chopped nuts (optional)

Method of Preparation:

1. Wash the quinoa
2. After rinsing, simmer quinoa in almond milk until it's cooked.
3. If preferred, garnish with chopped nuts, a drizzle of honey or maple syrup, and a mixture of berries.

LUNCH

Broiled Chicken with Roasted Potatoes

Preparation Time: 1 Hour

Serves: 4

Calories: 300 **Sugar:** 2g **Sodium:** 300mg

Ingredients:

Chicken breasts (4)

Potatoes (4 medium-sized, diced)

Olive oil (2 tablespoons)

Garlic powder (1 teaspoon)

Paprika (1 teaspoon)

Salt and pepper to taste

Method of Preparation:

1. Warm up the oven and grill.

2. Garlic powder, paprika, salt, and pepper are used to season chicken.

3. Put the potatoes on a baking sheet and the chicken on a grill pan.

4. Apply some olive oil to the potatoes and chicken.

5. To ensure doneness, broil chicken for 6-8 minutes on each side.

6. Bake potatoes in the oven until they become soft and brown.

7. On top of roasted potatoes, serve chicken.

Quinoa Salad with Edamame and Sweet Potatoes

Preparation Time: 40 Minutes

Serves: 4

Calories: 300 **Sugar:** 2g **Sodium:** 250mg

Ingredients:

Quinoa (1 cup, cooked)

Edamame (1 cup, shelled)

Sweet potatoes (2 medium-sized, diced and roasted)

Cherry tomatoes (1 cup, halved)

Cucumber (1, diced)

Red onion (1/2, finely chopped)

Olive oil (3 tablespoons)

Lemon juice (2 tablespoons)

Salt and pepper to taste

Method of Preparation:

1. Follow the directions on the package to cook the quinoa.
2. Quinoa, edamame, roasted sweet potatoes, cherry tomatoes, cucumber, and red onion should all be combined in a big bowl.
3. Mix the olive oil, lemon juice, salt, and pepper in a small bowl.
4. Over the salad, drizzle with the dressing and toss to mix.

Veggie Toast with Hummus

Preparation Time: 15 Minutes

Serves: 4

Calories: 400 **Sugar:** 1g **Sodium:** 300mg

Ingredients:

Whole-grain bread slices (4)

Hummus (1 cup)

Avocado (1, sliced)

Cherry tomatoes (1 cup, sliced)

Cucumber (1, sliced)

Radishes (4, thinly sliced)

Sprouts (1 cup)

Salt and pepper to taste

Method of Preparation:

1. Toast the slices of wholegrain bread.
2. Cover each slice evenly with hummus.
3. Add sliced avocado, sprouts, cucumber, radishes, and cherry tomatoes on top.
4. To taste, add salt and pepper for seasoning.

Salmon with Roasted Vegetables

Preparation Time: 30 minutes

Servings: 4

Calories: 350 **Sugar:** 2g **Sodium:** 150mg

Ingredients:

4 salmon fillets

2 cups broccoli florets

1 red bell pepper, sliced

1 zucchini, sliced

2 tablespoons olive oil

1 teaspoon garlic powder

Salt and pepper to taste

Method of Preparation:

1. Set oven temperature to 400°F, or 200°C.
2. Salmon fillets should be put on a baking pan.

3. Combine the bell pepper, zucchini, and broccoli in a bowl and toss with the olive oil, salt, pepper, and garlic powder.

4. Surround the salmon on the baking sheet with the vegetable mixture.

5. Bake for 20 to 25 minutes, or until the veggies are soft and the salmon is cooked through.

6. Arrange the vegetables on top of the cooked salmon.

Grilled Turkey Sandwich with Cottage Cheese

Preparation Time: 20 minutes

Servings: 4

Calories: 400 **Sugar:** 4g **Sodium:** 600mg

Ingredients:

8 slices gluten-free bread

1 lb. turkey breast, sliced

1 cup arugula

1 tomato, sliced

4 tablespoons Dijon mustard

1 cup low-fat cottage cheese

Method of Preparation:

1. Set a grill or grill pan to preheat.
2. Cook slices of turkey on a grill until done.
3. Toast the slices of gluten-free bread.
4. Drizzle each slice with Dijon mustard.
5. Put tomato slices, rocket and cooked turkey on sandwiches.
6. Serve with low-fat cottage cheese on the side.

Baked Tilapia with Quinoa Pilaf

Preparation Time: 40 minutes

Servings: 4

Calories: 300 **Sugar:** 2g **Sodium:** 200mg

Ingredients:

4 tilapia fillets

1 cup quinoa, rinsed

2 cups chicken or vegetable broth

1 onion, finely chopped

1 bell pepper, diced

2 cloves garlic, minced

1 teaspoon cumin

Salt and pepper to taste

Method of Preparation:

1. Turn the oven on to 375°F, or 190°C.
2. Tilapia fillets are seasoned with cumin, salt, and pepper.
3. Tilapia should be baked in a baking dish for 15 to 20 minutes, or until the fish flake easily.
4. Sauté the onion, bell pepper, and garlic in a pot until they become tender.
5. To the pot, add the quinoa, broth, and cumin. After bringing to a boil, lower the heat and simmer the quinoa until it is tender.
6. Tilapia should be served atop quinoa pilaf.

Cauliflower Rice Bowl with Chickpeas and Spinach

Preparation Time: 30 Minutes

Serves: 4

Calories: 295 **Sugar:** 41g **Sodium:** 785mg

Ingredients:

1 (15-ounce can) Chickpeas

1 tablespoon Olive Oil

1 teaspoon Chili Powder

1/2 teaspoon Garlic Powder

1/2 teaspoon Ground Cumin

Pinch of Sea Salt

Pinch of Brown Sugar

1 medium (5-6″ diameter) head Cauliflower

1 1/2 tablespoons Olive Oil

4 cloves Garlic, pressed or minced

1 medium (196g) Zucchini, diced

1 small (74g) Green Bell Pepper, diced

1 cup frozen corn, defrosted

2 teaspoon Chili Powder

1/2 teaspoon Pepper

1/2 teaspoon Cumin

1 teaspoon Salt

1/2 tablespoon Lemon Juice

2 Plum Tomatoes

Method of Preparation:

Set oven temperature to 450°F (230°C).

Use silicone mats or parchment paper to line a baking sheet.

Combine all the ingredients for the roasted chickpeas in a medium-sized bowl.

Transfer the chickpeas onto the parchment paper-lined baking sheet, and bake for 20 to 22 minutes, tossing them once after 12 minutes.

They are ready to be removed from the oven when they seem shriveled and browned.

As the chickpeas roast, chop the cauliflower into chunks and pulse it in a food processor in batches or grate it by hand until it resembles rice.

With the remaining olive oil, heat a sauté pan over medium-high heat.

Add the minced garlic, stir, then add the bell pepper and zucchini. Sauté for two to three minutes, or until the garlic starts to brown.

Sauté the maize kernels for a further two to three minutes.

When the cauliflower is just soft, add the spices (ground cumin, cayenne pepper, chili powder, and salt) and simmer for a further two to three minutes.

Move the vegetable mixture into a sizable serving dish.

Add the chopped tomatoes, chickpeas, and lemon juice and stir gently.

If desired, garnish with sliced avocado or cilantro.

Carrot and Couscous Soup

Preparation Time: 1 Hour

Serves: 6

Calories: 170 **Sugar:** 8g **Sodium:** 958mg

Ingredients:

2 tablespoons olive oil

4 garlic cloves, chopped

1 large yellow onion, chopped

6 large red bell peppers, chopped into 1-inch pieces

4-5 large carrots (about 1 lb.), thinly sliced or chopped

1 teaspoon ground cumin

1/2 teaspoon sweet paprika

3 cups chicken or vegetable broth

1 teaspoon kosher salt

1 tablespoon prepared harissa

handful of chopped parsley

Couscous

1/2 cup chicken or vegetable broth

1/2 cup dried fine couscous

Method of Preparation:

1. In a big pot, warm up the olive oil over medium heat.

2. Add chopped onion and garlic, and sauté for approximately 5 minutes, stirring now and again, until lightly browned.

3. Cook the carrots for an additional four to five minutes, stirring them regularly.

4. Add the bell peppers and simmer for about five minutes, or until soft.

5. Add the salt, paprika, and cumin after adding the stock.

6. When the vegetables are extremely soft, bring to a boil, lower the heat to low, cover, and simmer for 20 to 25 minutes.

7. Make the couscous while the vegetables are cooking.

8. Heat the broth in a small saucepan over medium-high heat until it boils.

9. After removing from the heat, stir in the couscous, cover, and keep it somewhere warm for at least five to ten minutes.

10. Once the vegetables are soft, transfer the soup to a blender or use an immersion blender to purée it right in the pot.

11. Add salt to taste and stir in the harissa.

12. Spoon soup into bowls. Using a fork, fluff the couscous and mix it into the broth.

Zucchini Noodles with Kale and Tomato Sauce

Preparation Time: 30 Minutes

Serves: 5

Calories: 400 **Sugar:** 1g **Sodium:** 300mg

Ingredients:

8oz - Dried Pasta

1 Tbsp - Coconut Oil

1/2 - Onion

4 Cloves - Garlic

2 - Small Zucchini's, Chopped

3 Cup - Kale, Chopped

1 Cup - Vegetable Broth

2.5 Cups - Tomato Sauce

1 Cup - Vegan Milk

1 Tbsp - Italian Spice Blend (oregano, thyme, rosemary, etc)

1 tsp - Paprika

1/2 tsp - Cayenne Pepper (for an added kick!)

Sea Salt and Black Pepper to taste

OPTIONAL - Chopped Parsley, Kalamata Olives, and Vegan Cheese to garnish!

Method of Preparation:

1. Start by slicing all of your vegetables (the kale should be sliced into bite-sized pieces, and the zucchini can be diced into slices that are 1 centimeter broad).

2. Heat up some water in a pot for your pasta.

3. Observe the directions found on the packaging.

4. After it's done, drain and reserve.

5. Heat a pot with oil, onions, and garlic over medium heat. Simmer for three to five minutes.

6. Stir in the kale, zucchini, and vegetable broth.

7. Simmer and cover for three minutes.

8. Now add the seasonings, vegan milk, and tomato sauce.

9. Cook, stirring, over medium-low heat.

10. After the kale and zucchini are cooked to your preference and have softened enough to pierce with a fork, remove from the heat and combine your cooked

Lentil Tacos with Avocado

Preparation Time: 40 Minutes

Serves: 9

Calories: 400 **Sugar:** 2g **Sodium:** 450mg

Ingredients:

1 batch zesty lentils (see below)

2 ripe avocados, peeled, pitted, and diced

1 large handful fresh baby arugula

1 cup roughly-chopped fresh cilantro leaves

quarter of a small red onion, peeled and thinly-sliced

1 tablespoon fresh lime juice

(optional) 1 serrano pepper, thinly sliced

corn or flour tortillas

(optional) crumbled cotija cheese or queso fresco

1 cup uncooked black (beluga) or green (French) lentils

2.5 cups vegetable or chicken stock

1/2 teaspoon garlic powder

1/2 teaspoon ground cumin

pinch of salt and black pepper

Method of Preparation:

1. Make the lentils according to the recipe below.
2. Put away.

3. Avocado, rocket, cilantro, red onion, lime juice and Serrano pepper (if using) should all be combined in a big bowl.

4. Gently toss until well blended.

5. Fill your tortillas with lentils, top with avocado mixture, and garnish with shredded cheese (if using) to assemble the tacos.

6. To prepare the lentils, rinse them in a fine-mesh strainer with water, making sure to remove and dispose of any small stones that may have found their way in.

7. After transferring the lentils to a medium-sized saucepan, mix in the stock, ground cumin, garlic powder, salt, and pepper.

8. Bring the mixture to a boil over medium-high heat.

9. Once the lentils are soft, reduce heat to medium-low and simmer for 20 to 25 minutes, stirring periodically.

DINNER

Broccoli Quinoa Patties with Almond Butter

Preparation Time: 20 minutes

Serves: 4

Calories: 300 **Sugar:** 2g **Sodium:** 200mg

Ingredients:

2 cups cooked quinoa

2 cups finely chopped broccoli

1/2 cup almond butter

1/4 cup grated Parmesan cheese

2 eggs

1 teaspoon garlic powder

Salt and pepper to taste

Olive oil for cooking

Method of Preparation:

1. Quinoa, chopped broccoli, almond butter, Parmesan cheese, eggs, garlic powder, salt, and pepper should all be combined in a big bowl.
2. Blend the ingredients until they are properly blended.
3. Patties should be formed out of the batter and put on a baking sheet with liners.
4. In a skillet over medium heat, warm the olive oil.
5. Cook until golden brown, 3–4 minutes per side for the patties.
6. Warm up and serve.

Roasted Vegetable Sandwich with Hummus

Preparation Time: 30 minutes

Serves: 4

Calories: 250 **Sugar:** 3g **Sodium:** 180mg

Ingredients:

1 zucchini, sliced

1 red bell pepper, sliced

1 yellow bell pepper, sliced

1 red onion, sliced

2 tablespoons olive oil

Salt and pepper to taste

8 slices gluten-free bread

Hummus for spreading

Method of Preparation:

1. Set oven temperature to 400°F, or 200°C.
2. Add olive oil, salt and pepper to the zucchini, red and yellow peppers and red onion.
3. Bake the veggies for 20 to 25 minutes, or until they are soft.
4. Toast the slices of gluten-free bread.
5. Drizzle each slice with hummus and garnish with roasted veggies.
6. Place the sandwiches together and serve.

Curried Chickpea Wraps

Preparation Time: 25 minutes

Serves: 4

Calories: 320 **Sugar:** 4g **Sodium:** 220mg

Ingredients:

2 cans chickpeas, drained and rinsed

2 tablespoons olive oil

2 teaspoons curry powder

1 teaspoon ground cumin

1/2 teaspoon turmeric

Salt and pepper to taste

1 cup shredded cabbage

1/2 cup plain Greek yogurt

4 gluten-free tortillas

Method of Preparation:

1. Heat the olive oil in a pan over medium heat.
2. Stir in chickpeas, cumin, turmeric, curry powder, salt, and pepper.
3. Cook, stirring periodically, for 5 to 7 minutes.

4. Combine Greek yoghurt and shredded cabbage in a
   bowl.

5. Warm up the tortillas without gluten.

6. Spread the chickpea mixture over each tortilla, then
   top with the cabbage-yogurt mixture to assemble the
   wraps.

7. After rolling, serve the wraps.

Avocado Veggie Sandwich

Preparation Time: 10 minutes

Serves: 1

Calories: 300 **Sugar:** 2g **Sodium:** 300mg

Ingredients:

2 slices gluten-free bread

1/2 avocado, mashed

1/4 cup cucumber, thinly sliced

1/4 cup bell pepper, thinly sliced

1/4 cup cherry tomatoes, sliced

1/4 cup alfalfa sprouts

Salt and pepper to taste

Method of Preparation:

1. Toast the gluten-free bread slices.
2. Spread mashed avocado on one side of each slice.
3. Layer cucumber, bell pepper, cherry tomatoes, and alfalfa sprouts on one slice.
4. Sprinkle with salt and pepper.
5. Top with the second slice to create a sandwich.
6. Cut in half and serve.

Grilled Fish Tacos with Avocados

Preparation Time: 20 minutes

Serves: 2

Calories: 350 **Sugar:** 1g **Sodium:** 200mg

Ingredients:

2 tilapia fillets

1 tablespoon olive oil

1 teaspoon cumin

1 teaspoon paprika

1/2 teaspoon garlic powder

Salt and pepper to taste

4 gluten-free corn tortillas

1 cup shredded cabbage

1 avocado, sliced

Fresh cilantro for garnish

Method of Preparation:

1. Heat the grill.
2. Combine garlic powder, cumin, paprika, olive oil, salt, and pepper. Coat the fillets of tilapia.
3. To ensure doneness, grill fish for 3–4 minutes on each side.
4. Grilled tortillas are warm.
5. Fill tortillas with flake fish. Add some cilantro, avocado slices, and shredded cabbage on top.

Stir-Fried Shrimp and Vegetables

Ingredients:

1 pound shrimp, peeled and deveined

2 tablespoons olive oil

2 cups broccoli florets

1 bell pepper, sliced

1 carrot, julienned

2 cloves garlic, minced

1 tablespoon ginger, grated

2 tablespoons gluten-free soy sauce

1 tablespoon rice vinegar

1 teaspoon sesame oil

Green onions for garnish

Method of Preparation:

1. Warm up some olive oil in a skillet or wok.
2. Stir-fry the prawns until they turn pink.
3. Take out of the pan.
4. Once the veggies are soft, stir-fry the broccoli, bell pepper, carrot, garlic, and ginger.
5. Reintroduce the rice vinegar, sesame oil, soy sauce and prawns.

6. To mix, toss.

7. Serve with green onions as a garnish.

Quinoa and Roasted Vegetables

Preparation Time: 50 minutes

Serves: 6

Calories: 233 **Sugar:** 3g **Sodium:** 300mg

Ingredients:

1 medium red onion, thickly sliced

2 medium sliced zucchinis

2 bell peppers (yellow or red), sliced

2 carrots, peeled and sliced

6-8 whole cloves garlic, peeled

3 ½ tablespoons olive oil, divided use

1 tablespoon fresh thyme (or 1 teaspoon dried)

Kosher salt

Black pepper

1 cup quinoa

2 cups low sodium vegetable or chicken stock

1 tablespoon balsamic vinegar

½ teaspoon Dijon mustard

Method of Preparation:

1. Turn the oven on to 425°F.
2. Arrange the bell peppers, onions, zucchini, carrots, and garlic on a big roasting pan.
3. Pour in a quarter of a cup of olive oil. Add a sprinkling of thyme and season with a little salt and pepper.
4. Roast the vegetables for 30 to 35 minutes, or until they are tender and caramelised.
5. Halfway through, if you are using two baking sheets, rotate the pans.
6. Make the quinoa while the vegetables are roasting.
7. In a medium saucepan, combine the quinoa and vegetable (or chicken) stock; place over high heat and bring to a boil.
8. Turn down the heat to low and cover the pot. Simmer for 12–15 minutes, or until done.

9. Add salt to taste to season.

10. Take the quinoa off the stove and place it in a big bowl.

11. To the bowl, add the roasted vegetables.

12. In a small bowl, whisk together the balsamic vinegar, Dijon mustard, and the remaining 2 tablespoons olive oil.

13. After adding the dressing, toss the grains and veggies to mix them together.

14. Warm or cool, serve.

Brown Rice Pilaf

Preparation Time: 45 minutes

Serves: 6

Calories: 250 **Sugar:** 2g **Sodium:** 200mg

Ingredients:

1 tablespoon olive oil

1 small yellow onion, chopped

3 garlic cloves, minced

1 cup long grain brown rice (not instant)

2 1/2 cups fat-free low-sodium chicken broth or 2 1/2 cups vegetable broth

salt & pepper, to taste

Method of Preparation:

1. Heat the oil in a small skillet over medium-high heat.
2. Add the onion and garlic, and stir-fry for about 5 minutes, or until the onion turns golden.
3. For one minute, add the rice and sauté.
4. Bring the broth to a boil after adding it and seasoning with salt and pepper to taste.
5. Shut off the heat and cover.
6. Simmer for 45 to 50 minutes, or until the rice is soft and most of the liquid has been absorbed.
7. Periodically check the rice and add more water if needed.
8. Before serving, uncover the rice and let it stand for five minutes.

Lentil Soup

Preparation Time: 45 minutes

Serves: 8

Calories: 311 **Sugar:** 4g **Sodium:** 111mg

Ingredients:

2 tbsp olive oil

1 onion, chopped

2 garlic cloves, minced

1 large carrot , chopped

2 celery ribs , chopped

2 cups / 400g dried lentils

400g / 14 oz crushed tomato

 6 cups vegetable or chicken stock / broth, low sodium

1/2 tsp each cumin and coriander powder

1 1/2 tsp paprika powder

2 dried bay leaves

1 lemon (zest + juice)

1/4 tsp salt and pepper, each

Chopped fresh parsley, for garnish

Warm bread, to serve

Method of Preparation:

1. Heat oil in a large pot over medium heat.

2. Add garlic and onion, cook for 2 minutes.

3. Add celery and carrot.

4. Cook for 7 - 10 minutes or until softened and the onion is sweet.

5. Don't rush this step, it is key to the flavour base of the soup.

6. Add all remaining ingredients except the lemon and salt. Stir.

7. Increase heat and bring to simmer.

8. Scoop scum on the surface off and discard (do this again during cooking if required).

9. Place lid on and turn heat down to medium low.

10. Simmer for 35 - 40 minutes or until lentils are soft.

11. Remove bay leaves.

12. To thicken the soup, use a stick blender, do 2 or 3 quick whizzing.

13. Add a touch of water if you want to adjust soup consistency.

14. Season to taste with salt and pepper.

15. Grate over the zest of the lemon then add a squeeze of lemon juice just before serving.

16. Garnish with parsley if desired and serve with warm crusty bread slathered liberally with butter!

Egg White Omelet

Preparation Time: 25 minutes

Serves: 2

Calories: 120 **Sugar:** 1g **Sodium:** 200mg

Ingredients:

8 egg whites

1 teaspoon sea salt

½ teaspoon ground black pepper

2 tablespoons avocado oil

¼ medium onion, thinly sliced

½ medium red bell pepper, thinly sliced

½ medium zucchini, thinly sliced

2 cloves garlic, thinly sliced

4 slices crispy bacon; crumbled (optional)

¼ cup grated parmesan (optional)

Method of Preparation:

1. Beat the egg whites, ground pepper, and half a teaspoon of sea salt together in a medium-sized bowl until foamy.
2. In a big skillet, warm the avocado oil over medium-high heat.
3. Add the bell pepper, onion, and half a teaspoon of sea salt. Sauté for three minutes, or until the vegetables start to soften.
4. For about three more minutes, add the zucchini and garlic and sauté until the zucchini starts to soften.
5. Scatter the egg white mixture over the vegetables, tilting the pan so that the eggs get into all the crevices.
6. Reduce the temperature.
7. Once the egg whites are no longer transparent, simmer them for three to five minutes while covered.
8. Lift the cover and turn the omelette over.
9. To make things easier, use two spatulas.

10. As an alternative, you may cover the skillet with a sizable dish board, flip the omelette onto it, and then slide it back into the pan.

11. Simmer for one more minute.

12. If using, coat half of the eggs with the grated parmesan and bacon.

13. To form a half-moon, fold the omelette over the cheese and bacon.

14. Once the heat is off, cover the dish and leave it for one to two minutes, or until the cheese has melted. You can skip this step and serve immediately if you decide not to add the bacon or parmesan.

15. Once cut in half, serve.

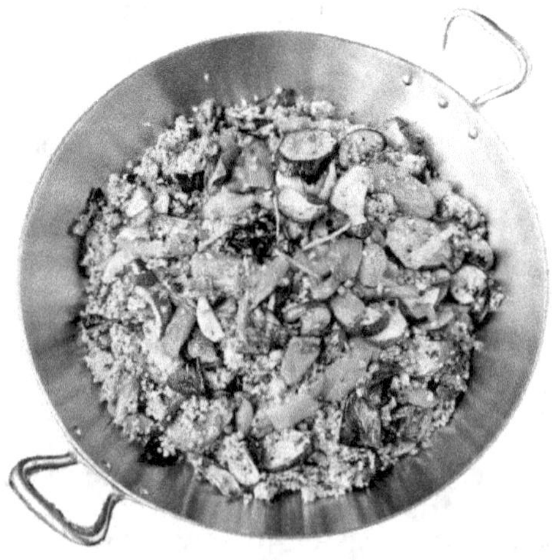

CONCLUSION

In conclusion, it is critical to follow a well-planned diet in order to effectively manage cirrhosis and fatty liver disease.

This dietary strategy in this book seeks to improve your general health, lessen hepatic stress, and possibly even halt the advancement of certain disorders.

You can enhance your general health and liver function by consuming fewer drugs and increasing your consumption of nutrient-dense, whole foods.

The focus on including lean proteins, whole grains, and a variety of vibrant fruits and vegetables provide vital vitamins, minerals, and antioxidants that promote liver function.

Carefully weighing portion sizes contributes to weight management, which is essential for reducing the risk of fatty liver disease. It also helps control caloric intake.

Cutting back on sodium, saturated fats, and added sugars is essential to reducing liver strain and treating related issues. This meal plan explicitly targets the particular difficulties brought on by liver illnesses in addition to adhering to general health recommendations.

 Furthermore, maintaining proper hydration promotes a number of biological processes and facilitates the body's removal of pollutants.

If you are in the process of managing cirrhosis or fatty liver disease, you must adjust your diet to suit your unique requirements, taking into account any dietary sensitivities or underlying diseases.

Dietary decisions should be made in accordance with medical advice and individual health objectives when consulted with healthcare providers on a regular basis, including dietitians.

This all-encompassing dietary strategy is a useful tool in the quest for liver health. It's important to understand, though, that dietary modifications might not be enough to treat these liver disorders, and that receiving medical care is crucial.

You can significantly improve the overall quality of your life and promote the health of your liver by combining a complete healthcare strategy with a nutritious diet.